THE 2022s DESSERTS COOKBOOK

Malika B. Josephsen

Contents

1. HAZELNUT TART WITH CHOCOLATE CREAM 1
2. DULCE DE LECHE 5
3. APPLE PIE 9
4. BLUEBERRIES PIE 17
5. RHUBARB PIE 21
6. CREAM FRAÎCHE 25
7. TARTE AU CHOCOLAT 31
8. BROWNIES 35
9. COCOA BISCUITS AND PISTACHIO 39
10. APPLE AND CHOCOLATE CAKE 43
11. SHORTBREAD AND CHOCO COOKIES 49
12. COCONUT AND CHOCOLATE SCONES 53
13. BLUEBERRY AND WITHE CHOCOLATE CAKE 57
14. CHESTNUTCHOCO CAKE 61
15. ALMONDS AND COCONUT COOKIES 67
16. SQUASH ROASTED 69

17. ROASTED CASHEWS 71

18. BERRIES MUFFINS 73

Chapter One

HAZELNUT TART WITH CHOCOLATE CREAM

We never go without chocolate spread in our house, I confess. When we go shopping, my husband and son (in that order) make sure to pick up a reserve jar. This is the consequence of using this cream in baking: a deliciously nutty, yet equally creamy, tart.

FOR ONE TART PAN (DIAMETER: 9 12 IN / 24 CM)

CRUST: Preheat oven to 350°F.

1 2/3 cup flour (200 g)

1 teaspoon of salt

1 teaspoon of sugar

12 cup (100 g) chilled butter, sliced into small pieces

ice cold water, 13 cup (80 ml)

TO MAKE THE FILLING: Preheat oven to 350°F.

cornstarch, 2 tbsp

2 cups cream (470 mL)

chocolate spread, 5 oz (140 g)

1 teaspoon of salt

1 tsp cinnamon

3.5 ounces (100 g) coarsely chopped hazelnuts

ADDITIONALLY:

Beans for baking in the dark

1. To make the dough, combine flour, salt, and sugar. Add the butter and quickly whisk everything together until it's crumbly.

2. Pour in the water and stir everything together rapidly to form a dough. If it's too dry, drizzle in a tablespoon of water at a time until it holds together.

3. Refrigerate the dough for at least 12 hours after wrapping it in plastic wrap.

4. Preheat the oven to 345 degrees Fahrenheit (175 degrees Celsius).

5. Remove the dough from the refrigerator and flatten it evenly into a tart pan with a detachable bottom. Remove the excess dough from the edges and use a fork to puncture the bottom. Fill with beans and cover with parchment paper. Allow to cool

after blind baking for 20 minutes. Remove the beans and parchment paper from the pan.

6. To make the filling, whisk together 14 cup (60 ml) cream and cornstarch. In a pot, thoroughly combine the remaining cream, chocolate spread, salt, and cinnamon. After that, add the starch mixture. Bring to a boil, then reduce to a pudding-like consistency by stirring constantly. Then set aside to cool.

7. Spread the filling over the bottom of the tart and bake for 25–30 minutes at 300°F (150°C) with top and bottom heat. Allow to cool before placing in the refrigerator for 4 hours. Sprinkle with hazelnuts just before serving.

Chapter Two

DULCE DE LECHE

Homemade dulce de leche can be used not only on cookies (see p. 104), but also as a soft, sweet bed for bananas, which are put into this lovely little nest of a tartlet with whipped cream. Together, these ingredients form a fantastic tart team.

MAKES 6 SMALL TARTLETS OR ONE LARGE TART (9 IN / 23 CM)

CRUST: Preheat oven to 350°F.

1 2/3 cup flour (200 g)

1 teaspoon of salt

1 teaspoon of sugar

12 cup (100 g) chilled butter, sliced into small pieces

ice cold water, 13 cup (80 ml)

TO MAKE THE FILLING: Preheat oven to 350°F.

1 can (14 oz / 400 g) sweetened condensed milk

3 banana slices, peeled and sliced

2/3 cup cream + 1 tbsp cream (200 ml)

ADDITIONALLY:

Garnish with cocoa powder or cinnamon sugar.

1. Combine the flour, salt, and sugar in a sifter. Cut the butter into small pieces, melt it, and quickly combine everything until it is crumbly.

2. Add the water and immediately incorporate everything into a dough. If the mixture is too dry, add a tablespoon of water at a time until it comes together.

3. Refrigerate the dough for at least 12 hours after wrapping it in plastic wrap.

4. Preheat the oven to 375 degrees Fahrenheit (190 degrees Celsius). Place the dough in 6 tartlet pans after rolling it out thinly. Prick the bottom of the dough with a fork several times and bake for 15–20 minutes. Then set them aside to cool.

5. Preheat the oven to 430°F (220°C) for the filling. Cover a baking dish with aluminium foil and pour in the condensed milk. Then transfer it to a larger baking dish and fill it with boiling water to a height of 34 inches (2 cm). Preheat the oven to 120°F and bake everything for 12 hours. Then, on the tartlet crusts, spread the cooled milk cream.

6. Slice the bananas into quarters and place them on top of the caramel. Pipe the cream onto the banana slices after whipping it to stiff peaks. If desired, dust the tartlets with cocoa powder or cinnamon sugar.

Chapter Three

APPLE PIE

INCLUDING CRANBERRIES

The apples in this pie caramelise beautifully in the oven, creating a delicious flavour combination with the cranberries. If you still have some vanilla ice cream in the freezer and aren't sure what to do with it, here's how to make the perfect companion for it.

9 12 IN / 24 CM DIAMETER FOR 1 PIE PAN

CRUST: Preheat oven to 350°F.

1 2/3 cup flour (200 g)

1 teaspoon of salt

1 teaspoon of sugar

12 cup (100 g) chilled butter

ice cold water, 13 cup (80 ml)

TO MAKE THE FILLING: Preheat oven to 350°F.

granulated brown sugar, 34 cup (150 g)

3 tablespoons flour

1 tsp cinnamon

1 teaspoon of salt

4 peeled, cored, and thinly sliced apples

1 handful cranberries, fresh

1 tablespoon of butter

ADDITIONALLY:

Brown sugar granules for sprinkling

1. Combine flour, salt, and sugar in a mixing bowl to make the dough. Add the butter in chunks and mix everything together quickly until you have a crumbly mixture.

2. Add the water and knead everything into a dough (again, fast). If the mixture is too dry, add a tablespoon of water at a time until it comes together.

3. Refrigerate the dough for at least 12 hours after wrapping it in plastic wrap.

4. In the meantime, combine the sugar, flour, cinnamon, and salt for the filling. Mix in the apples and cranberries until the apples are completely coated in the sugar mixture.

5. Preheat the oven to 390 degrees Fahrenheit (200 degrees Celsius).

6. Remove the dough from the refrigerator and flatten it out into a circle slightly larger than the pie pan with the help of a rolling pin.

7. Gently press the dough into the pan, arrange the apple slices in a single layer on top, dot with small bits of butter, and season with granulated brown sugar to taste.

8. Pinch the dough's edges over the apples and bake the pie in the oven for 40–50 minutes.

Orange Ricotta Tart

Do you wish it was summer? Here's a little taste of summer in tart form. Please remember to store it in the refrigerator to keep it fresh. Also, patience is required because cooling must occur immediately after baking in order for this delightfully light, gently sweet ricotta and orange tart to gain its full taste.

FOR ONE REMOVABLE BOTTOM TART PAN (9 IN / 23 CM DIAMETER)

CRUST: Preheat oven to 350°F.

1 2/3 cup flour (200 g)

1 teaspoon of salt

12 teaspoon sugar

12 cup (105 g) chilled butter, cut into chunks

ice cold water, 13 cup (80 ml)

TO MAKE THE FILLING: Preheat oven to 350°F.

Ricotta, 7.4 oz (210 g)

12 cup sugar (100 g)

12 tablespoons flour

1 organic orange, 12 tbsp zest

two eggs

ADDITIONALLY:

Garnish with powdered sugar

1. Combine flour, salt, and sugar in a mixing bowl to make the dough. Add the butter and immediately mix everything together until crumbly. Form the dough into a ball after adding the water. Refrigerate for at least 12 hours.

2. Remove the dough from the fridge, stretch it out thinly, and use it to line the tart pan. Trim the edges and re-chill the dough by poking it with a fork several times on the bottom.

3. Preheat the oven to 345 degrees Fahrenheit (175 degrees Celsius).

4. To make the ricotta filling, whisk together the sugar, flour, and orange zest in a mixing dish, then put aside. Toss the eggs

with the ricotta mixture and beat for 5 minutes, or until foamy. Take the pan out of the fridge and evenly spread the filling over the dough. Then bake for 45 minutes (without opening the oven door, even if you're really inquisitive and your patience is wearing thin as soon as this smell wafts across the kitchen).

5. Allow to cool before refrigerating, and sprinkle generously with powdered sugar just before serving.

Pecan Pie with Maple Syrup

Our maple syrup usually ends up atop a stack of wonderful pancakes at our place. That is, for the first time, my husband's job. He can simply do a better job with those circular breakfast marvels. But this time I've abducted the maple syrup and added a North American twist to a delicious pecan pie. For the kitchen, a mini Indian summer!

PAN (DIAMETER 9 12 IN / 24 CM OR 10 14 IN / 26 CM) FOR 1 PIE

CRUST: Preheat oven to 350°F.

1 2/3 cup flour (200 g)

1 teaspoon of salt

14 teaspoon sugar

7 tbsp chilled butter, sliced into small pieces

ice cold water, 13 cup (80 ml)

TO MAKE THE FILLING: Preheat oven to 350°F.

three eggs

12 cup + 2 12 tsp sugar (110 g)

34 cup maple syrup (240 ml)

3 tbsp melted butter

1 teaspoon of salt

150 g pecan halves, 5.3 ounce

ADDITIONALLY:

For the counter, flour

1. Combine flour, salt, and sugar in a mixing bowl for the pie dough. Rub in the butter with your hands until it is crumbly. After that, add the water and process until you have a smooth dough. Keep cold for at least 12 hours after pressing somewhat flat.

2. Then, on a floured countertop, roll out the dough and set it in a pie tin. Remove any protruding edges. Refrigerate any leftovers.

3. Preheat the oven to 375 degrees Fahrenheit (190 degrees Celsius).

4. In a separate bowl, cream together the eggs and sugar for the filling. Mix in the maple syrup, butter, salt, and pecan halves thoroughly.

5. Take the pie pan out of the fridge and evenly spread the filling on the bottom. After that, bake for 45 minutes in the oven.

Chapter Four

BLUEBERRIES PIE

To me, this straightforward blueberry pie smells and tastes like summer. Fresh blueberries, which bubble up wonderfully while baking and turn the sweet crust purple, are one of my favourite ingredients.

1 RECTANGULAR TART PAN (13 314 X 4 12 IN / 35 X 11 CM, PREFERABLY WITH REMOVABLE BOTTOM)

CRUST: Preheat oven to 350°F.

2 12 cup flour + 1 tsp (315 g)

1 teaspoon of salt

1 teaspoon of sugar

34 cup + 1 tablespoon + 1 teaspoon (190 g) chilled butter, sliced into pieces

12 cup Plus 1 tsp ice cold water (125 ml)

TO MAKE THE FILLING: Preheat oven to 350°F.

Blueberries, 17.6 oz (500 g) (fresh or frozen, not thawed)

a third of a cup (150 g) of sugar

cornstarch, 3 tbsp

1 tsp cinnamon

1 organic lemon's zest

1 teaspoon of lemon juice

1 whisked egg

a smidgeon of brown sugar granulated

1. Combine the flour, salt, and sugar in a mixing bowl. Add the butter and quickly combine everything into a crumbly mixture.

2. Add the water and mix everything together rapidly to form a dough. Add a tablespoon of water at a time until it holds together if it's too dry.

3. Cut the dough into two equal pieces and lightly press them together. Refrigerate for at least 12 hours after wrapping in plastic wrap.

4. Roll out a thin piece of dough and place it in a tart pan, trimming the extra borders. Place the pan in the refrigerator after poking holes in the dough with a fork.

5. Preheat the oven to 375 degrees Fahrenheit (190 degrees Celsius).

6. Meanwhile, combine the blueberries, sugar, cornstarch, cinnamon, lemon zest, and lemon juice in a mixing bowl and set aside for 10 minutes to prepare the filling. After that, remove the prepared pan from the fridge and pour in the blueberry mixture. Then relax once more.

7. Roll out the second half of dough and cut out different shapes with a tiny cookie cutter in the meantime. Carefully place the dough on top of the blueberry filling and trim the edges.

8. Brush the pie with an egg wash and sprinkle with granulated brown sugar before baking for 50–60 minutes. Allow to chill for 1 hour before serving.

Pie made with strawberries

CREAM FRAÎCHE CREAM FRAÎCHE CREAM FRAÎCHE CREAM F

When you want to take a break from the oven, create this pie. Because before making its great arrival, this fresh strawberry dream is prepared in the refrigerator.

8 IN / 20 CM DIAMETER PIE PAN OR SPRINGFORM PAN FOR 1 PIE

Whole grain shortbread biscuits, 7 oz (200 g)

12 cup (100 g) melted butter

1 13 cup cream cheese (300 g) (full fat)

250 g crème fraîche + 1 cup + 2 tsp

2 tbsp sugar (25 g)

14.1 ounces (400 g) cleaned and cut into tiny pieces ripe strawberries

ADDITIONALLY:

1 tbsp (100 ml) cream + 13 cup

For decoration, a few attractively appealing strawberries

1. Finely grind the biscuits and combine with the melted butter in a mixing dish. Then spoon the mixture into the springform pan or pie pan and firmly press it down. Put the pan in the fridge to chill.

2. In a separate bowl, thoroughly combine the cream cheese and crème fraîche. After that, add the sugar and combine everything.

3. Carefully fold in the strawberries, then remove the pan from the refrigerator. Spread the cream cheese mixture evenly over the crust.

4. Refrigerate the pie for at least one night. Garnish with whipped cream and strawberries the next day, just before serving.

Chapter Five

RHUBARB PIE

It appears to be difficult, but it is actually quite simple. Because of the lattice, the deliciously sweet and acidic rhubarb-orange filling tickles the tongue on the first bite, revealing the pie's secret.

9 INCHES / 23 CM DIAMETER PIE PAN

CRUST: Preheat oven to 350°F.

2 12 cup flour + 1 tsp (315 g)

1 teaspoon of salt

1 teaspoon of sugar

34 cup + 2 teaspoons (190 g) chilled butter, cut into cubes

12 cup + 1 tbsp ice cold water (125 ml)

TO MAKE THE FILLING: Preheat oven to 350°F.

26.5 oz (750 g) cleaned and sliced rhubarb

12 cup sugar (300 g)

cornstarch, 3 tbsp

1 organic orange (juice and zest)

1 lightly whisked egg yolk

1 tablespoon brown sugar, granular

ADDITIONALLY:

For the counter, flour

1. Combine the flour, salt, and sugar in a mixing bowl. Add the butter and stir everything together quickly until it's crumbly.

2. Pour in the water and immediately incorporate everything into a dough. If it's too dry, add a tablespoon of water at a time until it comes together.

3. Cut the dough into two equal pieces and lightly press them together until they are flat. Refrigerate for at least 12 hours after wrapping in plastic wrap.

4. Remove 12 ounces of dough from the fridge, roll it out on a lightly floured countertop, and place it in the pan. Allow the dough to expand slightly beyond the pan's edge.

5. In a mixing bowl, combine the rhubarb, sugar, starch, orange juice, and orange zest, then pour into the pie pan.

6. Preheat the oven to 430 degrees Fahrenheit (220 degrees Celsius) on both the top and bottom racks.

7. Roll out the leftover dough to a size slightly larger than the pan and cut into 12 strips with a pizza cutter. Now, on the pie, put this dough out in a grid pattern (see p. 106). Seal the pie crust by tucking the edges under.

8. Drizzle the whisked egg yolk over the pie and top with granulated brown sugar. Preheat the oven to 350°F and bake for 1 hour. Allow time for the dish to cool before serving.

Chapter Six

CREAM FRAÎCHE

Because I've made peace with pears and now bake with them more frequently, the tart tatin variation is also more frequently seen sneaking out of my oven. "I made a TART TATAAHN OH POAAR," repeat after me. Isn't that lovely? A little more of the little French girl emerges in you. And it feels fantastic.

APPROX. 12 IN / 30 CM DIAMETER TART TATIN PAN OR OVEN-SAFE PAN

3 pears, tiny

a squirt of lemon juice

sugar, 34 cup (150 g)

3 tablespoons butter, sliced

1 puff pastry roll (not frozen!) from the refrigerated area

ADDITIONALLY:

1 cup crème fraîche (200 g) for serving

1. Preheat the oven to 390 degrees Fahrenheit (200 degrees Celsius).

2. Remove the seeds from the pears and quarter them. In a mixing dish, combine the lemon juice and 14 cup (50 g) sugar and leave aside.

3. Melt the remaining sugar in a small, oven-safe skillet or a special tart tatin pan over medium heat, stirring constantly. Once the sugar has dissolved, gently set the pear quarters on top of the caramel, round sides down, or in the shape of a star. Allow the pears to simmer for about 5 minutes after adding the butter.

4. Cut a circle out of puff pastry that is slightly larger than the pan's diameter. Place the puff pastry on top of the pears and trim the edges of the dough with a knife so that the pears are well encased. Cut a small cross in the middle of the dough to allow heat to escape. Then bake for 12 hours in the oven.

5. Remove the tart from the oven and let it aside for 5 minutes before gently removing it from the pan. The best method to do this is to lay a plate over the pan and swiftly flip it over so that hot caramel sauce does not run down your fingers.

6. The tart is now ready to be served with crème fraîche.

MY ADVICE

This dessert goes well with cream or ice cream.

NECTARINES, BERRIES, AND CREAM CHEESE FROSTING

What I like best about this tart is how vibrant it is. It can even be more vibrant if you want it to be. Cherries, plums, and apricots, to name a few. This tart can be adorned with whatever you can find in your garden or at the farmer's market.

1 RECTANGULAR TART FORM (13 34 IN X 4 12 IN / 35 X 11 CM, PREFERABLY WITH REMOVABLE BOTTOM)

CRUST: Preheat oven to 350°F.

1 2/3 cup flour (200 g)

14 cup ground almonds (25 g)

2/3 cup powdered sugar (80 g)

1 teaspoon of salt

12 cup + 12 tbsp (120 g) cut into pieces extremely cold butter

a single egg

TO MAKE THE FILLING: Preheat oven to 350°F.

2/3 cup cream cheese (150 g)

12 cup crème fraîche (120 g)

4 tbsp sugar powder

3 nectarines, peeled, rinsed, and sliced

berries to taste (or cherries, plums, apricots, or others)

ADDITIONALLY:

For the counter, flour

For the pan, use butter.

1. Combine flour, almonds, powdered sugar, and salt to make the dough. Rub in the butter with your hands until it is crumbly.

2. Next, add the egg and immediately incorporate everything into a smooth dough. Refrigerate for 1 hour after shaping it into a ball and wrapping it with plastic wrap.

3. Take the dough out of the fridge and stretch it out on a floured counter until it is slightly larger than the tart pan. Place the dough in the lightly buttered pan, press it in, and trim the edges. Refrigerate the pan, as well as the dough, for additional 12 hours.

4. Preheat the oven to 375°F (190°F) on both the top and bottom racks.

5. Prick the dough several times in the bottom of the pan with a fork and bake for 15–20 minutes. After that, set aside to cool completely.

6. In the meantime, make a creamy filling with cream cheese, crème fraîche, and powdered sugar using a hand mixer and chill for 1 hour.

7. Pour the filling onto the dough, scatter the nectarine slices and berries on top, and serve the pie right away.

Chapter Seven

TARTE AU CHOCOLAT

Chocolate Paradise

My favourite beans are certainly cocoa beans. Here's to the Maya who grew them and the seafarers who carried them to Europe in brown gold. Because it has the ability to melt us in a variety of ways: fruit dipped in chocolate, chocolate-infused cakes, chocolate tarts, and biscuits. Chocolate is the common thread that binds all of these disparate dishes together. It's something that may truly offer people joy, and I know that with this component in the cupboard, I'll be prepared for any occasion.

WITH THE AID OF MERINGUE

This one is, in some ways, a wolf in sheep's clothing.
You envision cotton-soft clouds when you first look at the meringues, and you don't realise the chocolatey secret until after the fork has sunk into the chocolate sea—how exquisite!

FOR ONE REMOVABLE BOTTOM TART PAN (9 IN / 23 CM DIAMETER)

CRUST: Preheat oven to 350°F.

1 cup flour (125 g)

1 teaspoon of salt

12 cup (40 g) high-quality unsweetened cocoa powder

12 cup room temperature butter (115 g)

a third of a cup (60 g) of sugar

a single egg

3 tablespoons cream

TO MAKE THE FILLING: Preheat oven to 350°F.

chocolate spread, 4 tbsp

6.3 oz (180 g) coarsely chopped milk chocolate

80 g heavy cream, 13 cup

TO MAKE THE MERINGUE

Preheat oven to 350°F.

4 beaten egg whites

1 cup + 2 tbsp fine sugar (225 g)

1. In a mixing basin, combine flour, salt, and cocoa powder. In a separate bowl, cream together the butter and sugar, then add

the egg. A little at a time, alternate adding the flour mixture and the cream, and blend everything into a smooth dough. Wrap it in plastic wrap after lightly pressing it flat. Refrigerate for at least 1 hour before serving.

2. Preheat the oven to 345 degrees Fahrenheit (175 degrees Celsius).

3. Place the dough in the tart pan after rolling it out. Bake for about 20 minutes after poking it with a fork many times. Allow to cool completely before applying the chocolate spread.

4. In a double boiler, melt the chocolate with the heavy cream and set aside to cool for about 5 minutes. After that, spread this mixture on the bottom of the tart and chill for about 2 hours.

5. Just before serving, whisk the egg whites with the sugar until stiff, then distribute them over the cake. Make sure the entire surface of the chocolate is covered in egg white. Allow to brown for 5 minutes under a hot broiler. After that, serve and enjoy.

Chapter Eight

BROWNIES

GANACHE WITH RED WINE

This is another of my two men's all-time favourites. There is a nonalcoholic version for the little ones, but the brownies are finest fortified with a decent red wine in the ganache for the older ones.

FOR A 9 X 13 IN / 23 X 33 CM RECTANGULAR BAKING PAN

CRUST: Preheat oven to 350°F.

1 cup + 3 tbsp flour (150 g)

1 teaspoon of salt

2 tbsp cocoa powder, unsweetened and of good quality

Dark chocolate, finely chopped, 10.6 oz (300 g)

1 cup butter (230 g) cut into pieces

1 34 cup white sugar (350 g)

granulated brown sugar, 2/3 cup (125 g)

a dozen eggs

walnuts, chopped (3.5 oz/100 g)

FOR THE ANIMAL

dark chocolate, coarsely chopped, 8.1 oz (230 g)

a third of a cup (180 ml) of cream

30 g butter, 2 tbsp

1 tablespoon of red wine

ADDITIONALLY:

For the pan, use butter.

1. Preheat the oven to 345 degrees Fahrenheit (175 degrees Celsius). Line the bottom of the baking pan with parchment paper and butter it.

2. In a mixing basin, combine flour, salt, and cocoa powder; set aside.

3. In a double boiler, melt the chocolate and butter together. Remove from fire, stir in the two types of sugar, and set aside to cool.

4. Carefully fold three eggs into the chocolate mixture. Then add the remaining eggs and stir everything together until it

forms a uniform mixture. Under no circumstances should you over-stir the brownies; otherwise, they will become rock hard.

5. Fold in the flour mixture after sifting it over the chocolate. Do not combine. Only fold in until there are no more clumps of flour visible. Also, fold in the nuts for a few seconds. Then evenly distribute the dough in the pan.

6. Allow the brownies to cool after baking for 12 hours. They're a little soft, which is a good thing. That's a normal brownie texture.

7. Place the chocolate in a glass bowl for the ganache. In a small pot over medium heat, bring the cream and butter to a boil, then pour over the chocolate right away. Allow to rest for a few minutes before stirring gently to ensure that no air enters the ganache. The red wine should be mixed in before being spread on top of the brownies. Cut the brownies to the appropriate size once the ganache has hardened.

Tart with Chocolate Truffles

INCLUDING RASPBERRIES

The exact definition of dessert is this velvety-soft chocolate sin. It's not cooked, and it melts in your tongue as it slides off the fork. I especially enjoy topping it with fresh fruit.

6 IN / 16 CM DIAMETER FOR 1 SMALL SPRINGFORM PAN

8.8 oz (250 g) finely chopped high-quality dark chocolate

1 cup + 12 tbsp cream (250 ml)

1 tsp cinnamon

dusting cocoa powder

250 g raspberries, 8.8 ounce (or other berries)

1. Preheat oven to 350°F. Line a springform pan with parchment paper.

2. In a double boiler, melt the chocolate. In a saucepan, heat the cream and then remove it from the heat. Toss the cream with the chocolate and cinnamon. Stir until the mixture forms a smooth mass.

3. Pour the chocolate mixture into the springform pan and set aside for at least 4 hours in a cool location.

4. Toss with cocoa powder before serving, then top with fresh berries.

Chapter Nine

COCOA BISCUITS AND PISTACHIO

The pistachio tree is a deciduous tree that can reach a height of 12 feet and live for over 300 years. They are unmistakably determined. The pistachio, on the other hand, is a lovely component that gives these biscotti that extra crunch and flavour.

APPROXIMATELY 48 PIECES

2 12 cup flour (300 g)

1 tblsp baking soda

3 tbsp (30 g) high-quality unsweetened cocoa powder

175 mL (34 cup) vegetable oil

three eggs

1 cup + 2 tbsp sugar (225 g)

2 12 oz (70 g) unsalted shelled pistachios

1. Combine the flour, baking powder, and cocoa powder in a sifter and set aside in a bowl.

2. In a separate dish, whisk together the eggs and oil, then add the sugar. Gradually add the flour mixture, increasing the mixing speed as needed, until the dough is a homogeneous mass. Fold in the pistachios after that.

3. Wrap the dough in plastic wrap and place it in the refrigerator for at least 1 hour.

4. Preheat the oven to 345 degrees Fahrenheit (175 degrees Celsius). Using parchment paper, line a baking sheet.

5. On parchment paper, divide the dough into two pieces and roll each into a 12-inch (30-centimeter) long roll. Roll them out with a rolling pin until they're 3 in (8-9 cm) wide. Preheat the oven to 350°F and bake for 25 minutes.

6. Remove the baking sheet from the oven and lower the temperature to 300 degrees Fahrenheit (150 degrees Celsius).

7. Allow the rolls to cool almost completely before cutting into 12-inch (112-centimeter) thick slices. Then, on the baking sheet, lay them out flat next to each other and bake for another 15 minutes.

MY ADVICE

Pour melted chocolate over the biscotti if desired.

Blondies with White Chocolate

INCLUDING WALNUTS

Blondies are the name for white brownies. The blondes join together here, meet crispy walnuts, and thrill white chocolate fans.

SQUARE BAKING PANS (8 x 8 IN / 20 x 20 CM DIAMETER) FOR TWO

White chocolate, 5 14 oz (150 g), roughly chopped

a third of a cup (150 g) of butter

a third of a cup (150 g) of sugar

two eggs

1 teaspoon of salt

1 2/3 cup flour (200 g)

2 handfuls chopped walnuts

ADDITIONALLY:

For the pan, use butter.

1. Preheat the oven to 356 degrees Fahrenheit (180 degrees Celsius). Line the pan with parchment paper and butter it.

2. In a double boiler, melt the butter and chocolate. Allow to cool for a few minutes.

3. In the meantime, using a hand mixer, beat the eggs, salt, and sugar until frothy. After that, pour in the chocolate mixture.

4. Sift in the flour and stir thoroughly. Fold the walnuts into the mixture.

5. Pour the dough into the prepared pan and bake for about 12 hours. Allow to cool before cutting the blondies into squares.

Chapter Ten

APPLE AND CHOCOLATE CAKE

We love apples, and we'll make apple pancakes, applesauce, apple crumble, and a variety of apple cakes anytime our little, old, gnarly apple tree produces fresh fruit for us in the autumn. I made an apple-chocolate cake to add some apple-related variety to our diet (and my oven). This is my new favourite apple recipe—and favourite chocolate cake—and I'm going to lean really far out the window to share it with the world.

FOR ONE SPRINGFORM PAN (DIAMETER: 8 IN / 20 cm)

3 apples, tiny

a squirt of lemon juice

dark chocolate, 8.8 oz (250 g), roughly chopped

1 tbsp cream (160 ml) + 34 cup

3 distinct eggs

cornstarch, 4 tbsp

3 tbsp maple syrup or honey

3 tbsp hazelnut flour (almonds, walnuts, or others)

1 tbsp sugar (brown)

ADDITIONALLY:

For the pan, use butter.

1. Preheat the oven to 375 degrees Fahrenheit (190 degrees Celsius). Butter the rim of the springform pan and line it with parchment paper.

2. Peel the apples, remove the seeds and stems, dice, and season with lemon juice before setting aside.

3. In a mixing basin, combine the chopped chocolate. In a pot, bring the cream to a boil and quickly pour over the chocolate. Allow it to sit for a few minutes before stirring until it has thickened into a sinfully creamy and chocolatey mess.

4. Gently fold in the egg yolks. After the preceding egg yolk has been thoroughly mixed in, add the next one. Combine the cornstarch with the rest of the ingredients.

5. Whip the egg whites until stiff peaks form, then fold in the honey (or maple syrup). Mix in a third of the egg-white mixture with the chocolate dough until thoroughly combined. Fold in the rest of the egg white mixture gradually.

6. Place the dough in the pan, lay it out evenly, and top with the apples. Ground hazelnuts (or any other nuts) and granulated brown sugar are sprinkled on top.

7. Preheat the oven to 350°F and bake the cake for 35–40 minutes. After that, the cake should be moist, similar to a brownie, so don't overbake it.

8. Remove it from the pan after it has cooled slightly.

Cake with Red Velvet

The combination between the cocoa powder and buttermilk gave the cake its original red hue. We can now enhance that impression with food colouring to create a cake that seems as if it came straight out of a fairy tale.

FOR THREE SPRINGFORM PANS (8 IN / 20 CM)

TO MAKE THE DOUGH:

1 cup + 12 tbsp room temperature butter (250 g)

3 13 cup sugar (660 g)

6 quail eggs

30 mL red liquid food colouring (2 tbsp)

3 tbsp high-grade cocoa powder, unsweetened

3 cups flour (375 g)

250 mL buttermilk, 1 cup + 1 tbsp

12 teaspoon salt

1 teaspoon of baking soda

1 tbsp balsamic vinegar

FROSTING INSTRUCTIONS:

50 g room temperature butter (3 tbsp + 1 tsp)

12 cup room temperature cream cheese (100 g)

1 14 cup powdered sugar (250 g) + a little additional

ADDITIONALLY:

For the pans, butter and flour are required.

1. Preheat the oven to 340 degrees Fahrenheit (170 degrees Celsius). The springform pans should be butter and floured. Preheat oven to 350°F. Line the bottoms of the pans with parchment paper.

2. Using a mixer, beat the butter and sugar until frothy. Add the eggs one at a time.

3. Combine the food colouring and cocoa powder in a mixing bowl until smooth, then add to the dough.

4. Alternate adding flour and buttermilk, then season with salt.

5. Dissolve the baking soda in the vinegar and add to the dough. Now, evenly spread the dough among the three

pans and bake for approximately 25 minutes. Allow it cool completely before removing the cake layers from the pans.

6. To make the frosting, cream together the butter and cream cheese. Mix in the powdered sugar until everything is combined into a spreadable mixture. You'll have to stir a little longer for that, but don't give up; it'll happen! If the mixture is still too tough after a lot of stirring, add a little milk. If the mixture appears to be too liquidy, add more powdered sugar.

7. Spread frosting on the first layer of cake, then arrange the second layer on top and frost once more. Spread the icing around the sides and top of the cake once all three layers have been stacked. Keep refrigerated until ready to eat.

MY ADVICE

If you don't have three springform pans, you can bake the layers in one pan.

Truffles de chocolat

When I pass a chic bakery in my hometown, cute little chocolate balls always smile at me. Even yet, rolling them up oneself isn't that difficult. The best part is that you can flavour them whatever you like. Vanilla, espresso, chile, hazelnut liquor, cinnamon, and on and on... I went with cardamom in this situation. Those who dislike cardamom might simply cut it out or substitute something else they prefer.

APPROXIMATELY 30 TRUFFLES

8 oz. dark chocolate (225 g)

1 cup cream (250 mL)

1 tsp. cardamom powder

3 tbsp + 2 12 tsp butter (55 g)

Toss with cocoa powder

1. Chop the chocolate into very fine pieces.

2. Bring the cream, together with the cardamom, to a boil, then pour over the chocolate. Stir continuously until a creamy chocolate cream forms. Stir in the butter slowly.

3. Allow 15 minutes for the chocolate mixture to chill in the refrigerator. After that, slice out tiny balls with a teaspoon and chill for 1 hour.

4. Toss the chocolate truffles in cocoa powder to finish.

MY ADVICE

These delectable chocolate balls are simple to box and make a wonderful present for family or friends.

Chapter Eleven

SHORTBREAD AND CHOCO COOKIES

SALT OF VANILLA

Even though the word "Hello" isn't stamped on them, these delectable chocolate biscuits with delicate, contrasting vanilla salt say "Hello." But, just in case you forget to eat them all, I scribbled it on the cookies again, just to be safe.

THIS RECIPE MAKES 8 SHORTBREAD COOKIES

12 cup powdered sugar (60 g)

5 tbsp room temperature butter (70 g)

4 12 tbsp vegetable oil (60 g)

1 cup flour (125 g)

3 tbsp cocoa powder (unsweetened, high-quality)

1 teaspoon of salt

a smidgeon of vanilla salt to sprinkle

1. In a mixing dish, combine the sugar, butter, and oil.

2. Combine the flour, cocoa powder, and salt in a small mixing bowl before sifting into the butter mixture. Knead into an even dough with your hands and wrap in plastic wrap. Refrigerate for about 12 hours.

3. Preheat the oven to 320°F (160°C) in the meantime. Using parchment paper, line a baking sheet.

4. Roll out the dough into a 1-cm-thick circle, sprinkle with a pinch of vanilla salt, poke with a fork several times, and bake for 12 hours.

5. Remove the shortbread from the oven and cut it into eight equal pieces. Allow it to cool before serving.

MY ADVICE

Vanilla salt is available from a variety of spice shops, but it's also simple to make at yourself. Place the pulp from four vanilla pods on top of one cup of sea salt. Now, using a pestle or a spoon, rub the vanilla pulp into the salt and keep well packed.

Strawberries with a Chocolate Coating

WITH A DIFFERENT TAKE

Who said strawberries had to be individually wrapped in chocolate?

With that in mind, we'll take 8 or 10 strawberries at a time and do things a little differently this time.

At least 8 to 10 times more delectable!

MAKES TEN (12 OZ) CHOCOLATE-COVERED STRAWBERRIES (300 G).

Milk chocolate, 5 13 ounces (150 g)

Dark chocolate, 5 13 ounces (150 g)

8 strawberries, big

1. Use a cut-out piece of freezer bag to line a small loaf pan.

2. In a double boiler, chop both types of chocolate and melt them together.

3. Cover the bottom of the pan with a thin coating of chocolate.

4. Wash the strawberries, remove the leaves, and chop off the tops so they can stand on their own.

5. Arrange the strawberries on top of the chocolate in the pan and drizzle the remaining chocolate over them. Allow to set (perhaps in the fridge) until firm. Remove the chocolate-covered strawberries from the pan after that.

MY ADVICE

In the summer, serve the chocolate-covered strawberries ice cold.

Chapter Twelve

COCONUT AND CHOCOLATE SCONES

Delicious scones are a great way to start the day on a Sunday morning. Apart from that, they make a lovely addition to any breakfast or brunch table. These handy tiny snacks, which come in a coconut flavour, are also great to bring on picnics.

YIELDS 8 SCONES

2 13 cup flour + 12 tbsp flour (300 g)

brown sugar, 2 tbsp

1 tablespoon of baking powder

1 teaspoon of salt

12 cup cold butter (115 g) sliced into pieces

1 pound of chocolate chips (chopped chocolate or chocolate chips)

12 cup coconut milk (120 ml)

two eggs

ADDITIONALLY:

In order to knead the dough, you'll need flour.

coconut milk, 2 tbsp

3 tbsp sugar (brown)

1. Preheat the oven to 390 degrees Fahrenheit (200 degrees Celsius).

2. Combine flour, sugar, baking powder, and salt in a mixing bowl. Crumble everything together with your hands after adding the butter. Add in the chocolate chips now.

3. Combine the coconut milk and eggs in a mixing bowl and add to the flour mixture. Knead into an even dough with well-floured hands. Add more flour if the dough is too sticky.

4. On a baking dish coated with parchment paper, roll out the dough into a 12-inch (4-cm) thick circle and cut into eight pieces with a sharp knife. Sprinkle with sugar after basting with coconut milk. (Do not separate the eight pieces of dough; instead, place the entire piece of dough in the oven whole.)

5. Bake the scones for 15–20 minutes, then serve while still warm.

MY ADVICE

These would very certainly be topped with clotted cream if they were true Brits. However, you can eat them with marmalade, crème fraîche, softly whipped cream, butter, maple syrup, and so on. Alternatively, going completely natural is a great option.

Chapter Thirteen

BLUEBERRY AND WITHE CHOCOLATE CAKE

FROSTED WITH WHITE CHOCOLATE

You're looking for a delectable little cake to enjoy in the garden on a Sunday afternoon? So, there you have it. On the outside, there's a layer of sugary icing, and on the inside, there's a layer of delectable blueberries for a light, refreshing contrast. Set up some lawn chairs and a table outside, drape a tablecloth over the table, and relax.

FOR TWO 8 IN / 20 CM DIAMETER SPRINGFORM PANS

TO MAKE THE DOUGH:

3 2/3 cup flour + 3 tbsp flour (450 g)

12 tsp baking powder 3 12 tsp baking powder

1 teaspoon of salt

1 cup + 5 tsp room temperature butter (250 g)

2 14 cup sugar (450 g)

1 vanilla pod's pulp was scraped out

4 quail eggs

250 ml milk + 1 cup + 1 tbsp

Blueberries, 14 oz (400 g)

FROSTING INSTRUCTIONS:

high-quality white chocolate, 6 oz (170 g), roughly chopped

14 cup cream (60 ml)

1 cup room temperature butter (230 g)

1 cup + 2 tsp powdered sugar (125 g)

ADDITIONALLY:

For the pans, butter and flour are required.

2 tbsp blueberry marmalade to serve as a garnish

1. Preheat the oven to 355 degrees Fahrenheit (180 degrees Celsius). The pans should be brushed with butter and dusted with flour.

2. Sift flour, baking powder, and salt into a mixing basin and set aside for the dough.

3. Using a hand mixer, whip together the butter, sugar, and vanilla pulp. One by one, crack the eggs into the mixture.

4. Alternate kneading the flour mixture and the milk into the dough at this point.

5. Toss 3 tablespoons blueberries in flour (so they don't sink to the bottom when baking), then mix them into the dough carefully.

6. Evenly distribute the dough between the two pans and bake in the oven for 30–40 minutes. Allow to cool before removing from the pans.

7. In a double boiler, melt the white chocolate and cream for the icing. Allow to cool before adding butter and powdered sugar. Using a hand mixer, beat the ingredients until it is spreadable.

8. Spread a thin layer of frosting on top of the first layer of cake, then top with blueberry marmalade and the second layer of cake. Apply the remaining frosting to the top and edges of the cake, then top with blueberries.

Chapter Fourteen

CHESTNUTCHOCO CAKE

Sweet chestnuts aren't simply for warming your shivering limbs at Christmas markets. They're also great with chocolate, and they're a great addition to this dessert.

FOR ONE 9.5 IN / 24 CM DIAMETER SPRINGFORM PAN

Dark chocolate, 10.5 oz (300 g)

Sweet chestnut purée, 15.3 oz (435 g) (can)

12 cup crème fraîche + 1 teaspoon (150 g)

3 12 tbsp room temperature butter (50 g)

4 beaten egg whites

6 12 tbsp sugar (80 g)

6 tablespoons flour

ADDITIONALLY:

For the pan, use butter.

1. Preheat the oven to 300 degrees Fahrenheit (150 degrees Celsius). Line the pan with parchment paper and butter it.

2. Chop the chocolate coarsely, melt it in a double boiler, and set it aside.

3. Combine the chestnut purée, crème fraîche, and butter in a mixing dish.

4. Whisk the egg whites until stiff, then gradually add the sugar.

5. Combine the flour and chocolate in a large mixing bowl, then stir in the chestnut cream completely.

6. Gently fold in the balance of the beaten egg whites after mixing in 13 of them with the chocolate dough.

7. Pour the dough into the pan and knock it several times on the counter to spread it out evenly.

8. Bake the cake for about 50 minutes in the oven. Then set it aside to cool.

MY ADVICE

You can dust the cake with cocoa powder and serve it with vanilla ice cream if desired.

Cake in an Ice Box

A childhood favourite that I've spiced up with a peppermint twist. At least, that's what I thought until the kids loved it just as much as the adults did, and the entire cake was devoured in a matter of minutes.

PAN FOR ONE SMALL CHILDREN'S LOAF

(If using a regular-sized loaf pan, double the amounts)

dark chocolate, 3 oz (75 g), roughly chopped

milk chocolate, 7 oz (200 g), roughly chopped

14 chocolate chunks with a mint filling (i.e., Andes)

Copha 2.6 oz (75 g) (solidified coconut fat)

13 cup + 2 tbsp cream (100 ml)

8 g vanilla sugar (2 tsp)

Butter cookies, 4.4 oz (125 g)

1. In a medium-sized pot, slowly melt the chocolate, Copha, and cream. Allow the mixture to cool before adding the vanilla sugar.

2. Use plastic wrap or aluminium foil to line the loaf pan. Place a small amount of the chocolate mass in the bottom of the pan, then pile on cookies and chocolate in that order. Finish with a chocolate layer.

3. Put that gem of culinary gold in the fridge! Allow 6 hours for the icebox cake to chill and harden.

4. Remove the cake from the pan by flipping it over, removing the pan liner, cutting yourself a piece, and enjoying.

DOUBLE CHOCOLATE CHOCOLATE CHOCOLATE CHOCOLATE CHO

Cake with Cocoa

It was gone as soon as it came out of the oven. What happened to cause that? With two schoolmates staying at our place for a free afternoon, we had three hungry mouths to feed. “Did your mother bake again?” the boys continue to inquire.

FOR ONE MEDIUM BUNDT PAN

TO MAKE THE DOUGH:

1 34 cup flour + 2 tbsp flour (230 g)

5 tbsp high-grade cocoa powder, unsweetened

1 tablespoon of baking powder

1 teaspoon of salt

4 quail eggs

220 g sugar + 1 cup + 2 tbsp

1 quart (240 millilitres) milk

12 cup butter (125 g) split into pieces

TO MAKE THE GLAZE:

milk, 14 cup (60 ml)

milk chocolate, 7 oz (200 g), chopped

ADDITIONALLY:

For the pan, butter and flour are required.

For garnishing, 3.5 oz (100 g) milk chocolate

1. Line a baking sheet with plastic wrap or aluminium foil and preheat the oven to 355°F (180°C). The pan should be butter and floured.

2. Sift flour, cocoa powder, baking powder, and salt into a bowl and set aside for the dough.

3. Using a hand mixer, beat the eggs and sugar until the mixture is light and fluffy. Then completely blend with the flour mixture.

4. Simmer the milk and butter until the butter has melted over low heat. Stir this mixture into the dough until it forms a uniform consistency.

5. Place the dough in the prepared pan and bake for 20–25 minutes. (Test with a toothpick!) Remove the pan from the heat and set aside to cool.

6. To make the glaze, in a small pot, bring the milk to a boil, then remove from the heat and pour over the chopped

chocolate. Allow the mixture to sit for a few moments before stirring it again and carefully glazing the cake.

7. Melt the remaining chocolate in a double boiler and pour over parchment paper right away. Allow the chocolate to firm in the refrigerator by rolling the parchment paper up quickly and gently. You'll find gorgeous, wavy chocolate flakes as you unroll the paper. Use them to decorate the bundt cake.

Chapter Fifteen

ALMONDS AND COCONUT COOKIES

No one will be able to resist the delicacy of this biscuit. Almond and cheese combine to form delicious sweets that will make your tongue dance. Make this cookie in double or more portions when you have free time, then store in a jar with a lid. Indulge in a serving of this unique cookie during your snack time.

2 Yield

Time to prepare: 25 minutes

List of Ingredients:

- a quarter-cup of almond butter
- a quarter-cup of grated cheese
- 2 yolks of eggs
- 1 pound of almond flour

- 12 cup flakes de coco

Procedure:

1. Preheat the oven to 250 degrees Fahrenheit and line a baking sheet with parchment paper.
2. In a mixing bowl, combine almond butter and egg yolks. Using an electric mixer, whisk until smooth and well mixed.
3. Stir in the shredded cheese until it is completely mixed into the butter mixture.
4. Stir in the almond flour and mix with a wooden spatula until the mixture forms a dough.
5. Finally, add the coconut flakes to the dough and stir just until incorporated.
6. Roll the dough into small balls and squeeze each one until it resembles a coin.
7. Arrange the coins on the prepared baking sheet and bake for 20 minutes, or until the biscuits are faintly brown on top.
8. Remove it from the oven and place it on a cooling rack.
9. Once the cookies have cooled, put them in a jar with a lid and eat them whenever you like.

143 calories per serving, 1.1 g sugar, 3.8 g net carbs, 12.6 g fats, and 5.4 g protein

Chapter Sixteen

SQUASH ROASTED

Almost all women, particularly pregnant women, make significant attempts to improve their skin and hair. Butternut squash is a type of food that is said to be good for your skin and hair. Butternut squash contains a lot of vitamin C, which helps to moisturise your skin, prevent wrinkles, and promote hair development. Butternut squash, especially when consumed by a pregnant woman, aids in the development of the baby's brain and spinal cord. The butternut squash increases a pregnant woman's chances of having a healthy baby.

2 Yield

Time to prepare: 45 minutes

List of Ingredients:

- Butternut squash cubes (12 pound)
- 34 tablespoons olive oil

- 14 teaspoon cumin
- almond butter, 2 tbsp.

Procedure:

Preheat the oven to 400 degrees Fahrenheit and line a baking sheet with parchment paper.

2. Melt the almond butter in the microwave, then whisk in the olive oil and cumin.

3. Cut the butternut squash into wedges after peeling it.

4. Toss the butternut squash with the butter mixture and spread on the baking sheet that has been prepared.

5. Roast the butternut squash for 30 minutes or until it is soft.

6. When it's done, take it out of the oven and place it on a serving platter.

7. Finally, serve and enjoy.

Each serving has 197 calories, 3.4 grammes of sugar, 16.5 grammes of net carbs, 14.3 grammes of fat, and 4.8 grammes of protein.

Chapter Seventeen

ROASTED CASHEWS

Unsweetened

Cashews are safe to eat during pregnancy unless you have a nut allergy to them. Among other nuts, cashew is without a doubt the best provider of protein and lipids. It's also high in fibre, iron, vitamin K, and magnesium, all of which are beneficial to a pregnant woman. Overeating cashews, on the other hand, might lead to weight gain. As a result, it's best to eat this snack in moderation.

4 % yield

Time to prepare: 15 minutes

List of Ingredients:

- 34 cup cashews, uncooked
- 12 tbsp. extra virgin olive oil

Procedure:

1. Preheat oven to 375 degrees Fahrenheit and line a baking sheet with parchment paper.

2. Bake the cashews for 15 minutes after spreading them out on the prepared baking sheet.

3. Every 5 minutes, stir the cashews. Pay care to the cashew's doneness because it might burn rapidly.

4. When the cashew is done, take it from the oven and sprinkle it with olive oil. Toss everything together.

5. Serve in a serving dish or jar while watching a movie.

Each serving has 153 calories, 1.3 grammes of sugar, 8.4 grammes of net carbs, 12.5 grammes of fat, and 3.9 grammes of protein.

Chapter Eighteen

BERRIES MUFFINS

This low-sugar berry muffin won't make a pregnant woman feel bad. Berry is not only harmless but also beneficial to a pregnant woman. It contains potassium, which is necessary for blood pressure regulation. As a result, it may be said that berry reduces the risk of preeclampsia in pregnant women.

4 % yield

Time to Prepare: 30 minutes

List of Ingredients:

• a quarter-cup of coconut oil

2 eggs (organic)

• 1 cup yoghurt (almond)

• 1 teaspoon of orange zest

• 1 to 12 cup almond flour

• 34 teaspoon cinnamon

• 14 cup blueberries, chopped

• 14 cup cranberries, chopped

Procedure:

1. Preheat the oven to 375°F and line 8 muffin cups with paper liners. Remove from the equation.

2. In a mixing dish, combine almond flour, orange zest, and cinnamon. Mix thoroughly.

3. Break the organic eggs and set them in a separate bowl. Stir until the mixture is barely beaten.

4. Mix the beaten eggs with the coconut oil and almond yoghurt until fully combined.

5. Pour the liquid mixture over the dry ingredients and whisk until everything is well blended.

6. Stir in the blueberries and cranberries, then divide the mixture among the muffin cups.

7. Bake the muffins for 20 minutes, or until a toothpick inserted in the centre comes out clean.

8. When it's done, take it out of the oven and set it on a cooling rack.

9. Place the muffins on a serving plate and serve immediately.

10. Have fun!

Each serving has 252 calories, 4.7 grammes of sugar, 11.6 grammes of net carbs, 21.8 grammes of fat, and 5.4 grammes of protein.

CPSIA information can be obtained
at www.ICGtesting.com
Printed in the USA
LVHW060216160722
723616LV00015B/805

9 781804 768921